Breastfeeding 101
PREPARE FOR THE SUCK

By Michelle McKeown Poole MS, RN, IBCLC

Illustrations by Beth McKeown, BFA

Breastfeeding 101: Prepare for the Suck

ISBN -978-1-7345287-0-1

TABLE OF CONTENTS

INTRODUCTION

Hi, mom-to-be!

I know what you want: the perfect breastfeeding experience.

You've heard a ton about the perks of breastfeeding, plus, "it's easy and natural." And why shouldn't it be? You have boobs, and soon you'll have a baby. You'll put the baby on the boob and voilà, breastfeeding!

And in a perfect world, your baby will latch effortlessly to your perfect nipples, and your perfect milk supply will start to flow into his perfect mouth and then he will produce the perfect number of diapers full of perfectly colored poos. (Yes, there are right and wrong colors of poos, and you will be a baby poo expert after reading this book.)

Now while the above scenario is certainly possible, I've found that achieving the ideal breastfeeding relationship takes some time. It's normal for moms to struggle through the first weeks of breastfeeding. If they don't get help early, many of these moms quit much sooner than they had planned.

But this doesn't have to be you.

Now keep in mind, despite reading this book and a handful of others, taking a class, and lurking on mommy forums, when the time comes for your baby to get onto your breast, you will probably still feel like you have no idea what you're doing.

If you are like most new moms, you will wonder,

"Am I doing it right?"

"I don't have enough hands!"

and

"Is anything coming out?"

You might also wonder after a feeding,

"Uhhh, is it normal for my nipples to look like I've been nursing a baby rhinoceros?" (NO!)

Preparing for any big event in advance yields the best results, and breastfeeding is no different. This book will cover the basics in a fun and easy way, and help you feel confident and committed to your feeding choice.

And you have made a great choice! Most women who manage to overcome the initial breastfeeding hurdles go on to experience a truly beautiful, rewarding, and unique breastfeeding relationship with their babies.

A Quick Note About Language Choices:

Whether you're expecting a girl, a boy, or a "theyby", I've got you covered. When talking about the baby, I'll alternate using "he," "she" and "they."*

When referring to a baby who is being raised in a "gender creative" way, "they," "they're" and "them" are the preferred pronouns and not a grammar mistake. ☺

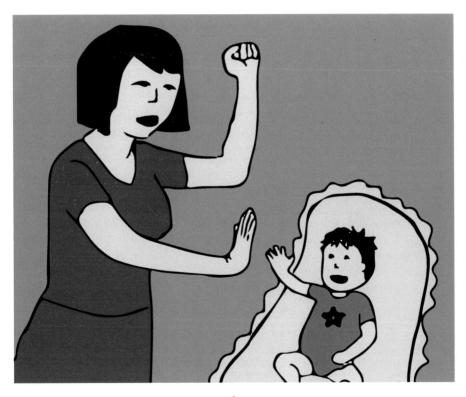

PART ONE: GET READY!

Take a breastfeeding class.

You've probably seen some photographic version of a mother breastfeeding her baby in a flowery meadow. This mom's freshly washed hair is blowing in the breeze, her makeup is flawless, her dress is white (I dare anyone to put on white clothing and keep it clean for more than 20 seconds while holding a baby), and sunbeams caress her blissfully breastfeeding baby. It is a scene that is beautiful, peaceful and even exudes a bit of a magical vibe. You can sense that this woman's nipples are not sore or blistered, that her baby is getting plenty of milk, and that he doesn't spit it up all over her shirt three minutes after he's finished.

But you know what? That image is a BIG FAT LIE!

Well, at least for the first few weeks.

Here's the truth: Breastfeeding tends to require time and hard work to become the easy and natural experience you're imagining. It takes practice, patience and usually at least a few days before you begin to feel like you know what you're doing. However, the more you know going in, the smoother your experience will be and the more quickly you will become an expert.

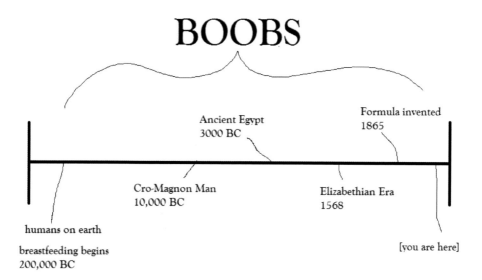

9

And of course for most women, breastfeeding does get easier after those first few days - otherwise the human race wouldn't be around! For hundreds of thousands of years, mothers have learned from other mothers and put in the work that delivered them to the Promised Land of Breastfeeding. In this wonderful world where breastfeeding is going well, a mom pops her baby onto the boob, baby eats, and that's that!

So to help you reach your goal of care-free happy breastfeeding, I encourage you to take a prenatal breastfeeding class. Now I'm not saying that by taking a class you'll avoid hardships. But understanding the challenges, preventing them if possible, and knowing when to get help will only make your life easier after the baby arrives.

And once you and your baby have it all figured out, you can go out into that meadow and have a photoshoot of your own.

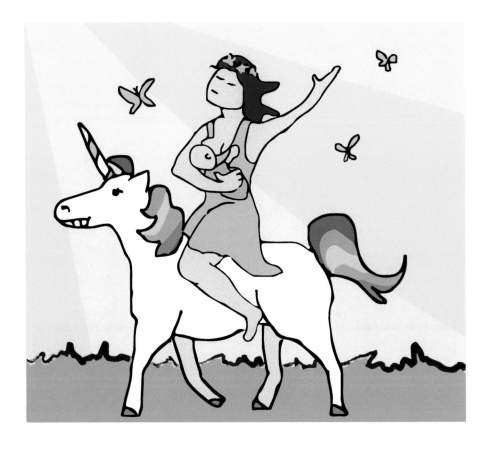

Talk to your support team.

Family and friends often wonder how they will be able to help with feeding if you've decided to breastfeed.

As a lactation consultant, I meet many families, and am always sizing up how their respective relationships are going to influence breastfeeding. The support people whom I know are going to be an asset to the feeding situation are the ones who sit on the couch glued to their phones while I help mom.

No, wait.

Those couch potatoes actually need to take a lesson from the support people who watch what I'm doing, follow my lead, ask a lot of questions, and sometimes even take pictures of what a comfortable deep latch looks like. Family and friends can help with latching the baby, getting you comfy once baby is feeding, making sure baby is eating well while latched, burping baby between sides, and putting baby down to sleep afterwards. Once breastfeeding is going well, many moms start pumping so that others can help by giving a bottle.

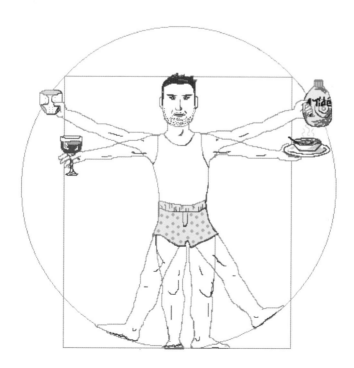

In addition to helping with feeding duties, there are many other ways the people around you can support your new family:

Doing Laundry: There will be lots of it. You will all start pondering why white is the standard color of a onesie. Why not black? Or at least yellow?

Cooking: While you are focusing all of your attention on feeding your baby, you may forget to feed yourself. Hopefully your people know their way around a kitchen...or at least know your favorite take out places.

Cleaning: You will cry tears of joy and profess your undying gratitude when you realize the dishes are done, the floor is swept and the bathroom is clean.

Holding the Baby While You Nap: This is a win-win situation, and you won't have to ask someone twice to snuggle with your newborn for a few hours (whereas you may have to ask them several times to clean your toilet).

So talk to your people about how they will be supporting your choice to breastfeed by helping out in a million other ways.

Buy stuff.

Technically, you only need your boobs and your baby to breastfeed. But if you have the means, there are a few items that will make breastfeeding more comfortable:

A good nursing pillow: You will be spending several hours a day nursing your baby, so get comfy! A firm foam pillow with built-in back support works wonders for the early days of breastfeeding.

Nipple butter/lanolin: This is for the first few days of normal soreness. Think of it as chapstick for your nips. But if your nipples are cracked, blistered, or bleeding, nipple butter isn't the answer. Beat-up nipples need professional breastfeeding help right away.

Good nursing bras: These should be supportive, easy-to-open with one hand, and not too tight. Some moms find that a regular (i.e. cheaper) front-fastening bra works just fine as a nursing bra.

An ergonomic baby carrier: If you have a baby who doesn't like to be put down (which is most of them), a carrier will let you move around and get stuff done while keeping baby happy. And as baby gets older and can self-attach to the breast, a good carrier will allow you to breastfeed discreetly and on-the-go.

Breast pads: Most moms leak for the first few days when their milk supply really starts to pick up. After that, there's really no telling what will happen on the leaking front. Some moms leak throughout their breastfeeding relationship, some leak occasionally, and some don't leak at all. A great initial plan is to have a box of disposable breast pads around, and then buy the reusable ones if you find you need them.

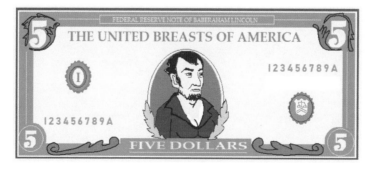

Meet prenatally with a lactation consultant.

Consider meeting prenatally with an IBCLC (International Board Certified Lactation Consultant) if:

- You have a history of endocrine or thyroid issues, diabetes, high blood pressure, PCOS, fertility concerns or if you suffer from a chronic health issue (these conditions may impact milk supply).
- You have had any kind of breast surgery.
- You have flat or inverted nipples (you can still breastfeed!)
- You were not able to reach your breastfeeding goals with a previous child.
- You are expecting multiples or a special needs baby.
- You have questions/concerns/anxieties about your breasts or breastfeeding.

PART TWO:
GETTING BREASTFEEDING OFF
TO A GREAT START

Skin-to-skin contact and the first "baby-led" latch.

A baby's first job in this world is to make a smooth transition from indoor living to outdoor living. He needs to start breathing, eating and maintaining his body temperature. These are all massive changes to the lifestyle your baby is currently accustomed to in-utero. But there is a very simple way you can make baby's new world much less stressful: Lay him on top of you!

In a skin-to-skin position, most babies:
- Stay warm
- Breathe more easily
- Have more regular heart rates
- Have more stable blood sugar
- Cry less
- Feed more often

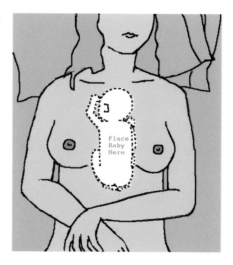

Skin-to-skin holding is the best way for your baby to transition to life on the outside. It helps all of his bodily systems perform at their peak and makes him feel at ease in this crazy new world.

But of course you're here to learn about breastfeeding, so let's focus specifically on how skin-to-skin contact and breastfeeding go hand-in-hand.

When baby is born, ask to have him placed on your chest, and only be removed if necessary during the first hour of life. Baby should be lying face down between your breasts, with his head turned to the side and covered with a blanket. Don't expect him to breastfeed right away. Your baby has a few things to do before latching on.

The first thing he will do is cry. You can't really blame him for that, since you'd cry too if you were suddenly and violently forced to leave your home through a chihuahua-sized doggy door. And crying is nature's way of allowing baby's lungs to fully open, so it is a truly beautiful sound.

Once he feels safe and secure on your chest, he'll calm down, and lie still and quiet with his eyes wide open, taking it all in.

Welcome to your new world, baby!

Soon, your baby will become more active. He'll lift his head, push himself up, and open and close his mouth. This activity will pick up until baby is making his way over towards one of your breasts. This is a total core body workout, so it's normal for him to take a few breaks.

Given time, he'll arrive at your nipple, and like a miniature Sherlock Holmes, start a serious investigation. Grabbing, rooting (turning his head from side to side) and tasting are all a part of his exploratory behaviors. Eventually, baby will feel satisfied that this is where dinner happens, and he'll dive in. Hopefully, he lands a nice deep latch and eats to his heart's content.

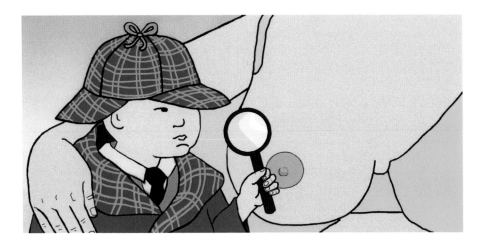

In most cases, all of this takes place within about an hour after birth. Your job during this first magical hour of life is to touch, talk to and gently guide your baby when needed. Let him know that he's got company in this thing. Relax and enjoy these amazing first moments with your baby.

(If your baby doesn't do these things, don't panic! Just keep him skin-to-skin and ask for help from the lactation consultant.)

The mother-led latch.

Hopefully you and your baby have a great first hour together and they show you they're already a pro when it comes to self-attaching. The laid back "baby-led" latch position is pretty awesome as it allows you to relax and be semi hands-free during a breastfeed. Plus, gravity tends to help your baby get a nice deep latch, and their hands help in the quest for the breast, rather than flailing around and getting in the way like they tend to do in mother-led positions.

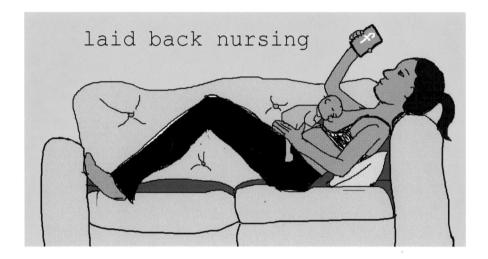

So if your first baby-led latch went well, congrats! Now you know that baby can get on the boob whenever you get into a reclined position.

But what about when you're out and about? Will you need to lie down on the mall bench and take your top off when baby needs to eat? Technically, the law says you're allowed to do this...but most moms prefer a more practical option, where they sit upright and take control of the latch.

Before we walk through a mom-led latch though, I'd like you to try two experiments to get you thinking about what your baby needs to look like when you latch him:

The Drinking Experiment: Turn your head all the way to the side and swallow. Comfortable? Now put your chin to your chest and swallow. Easy or hard? And while your chin is down in your chest, try to open it as widely as you can. Frustrating and difficult, right?

Now pretend to take a drink as you normally would. Notice your body position. Your ear, shoulder and hips are aligned, and your chin is slightly upturned.

The Eating Experiment: Imagine taking a bite out of a big sandwich. You squish the sandwich down in your hands so that you can fit your mouth around the whole thing. Next, you put the squished sandwich onto your lower jaw and then bring your upper jaw up and over the top of the sandwich in order to shove in as much as you can. (Well, ok, so maybe this is only when you're at home and no one is watching. But you get the point.)

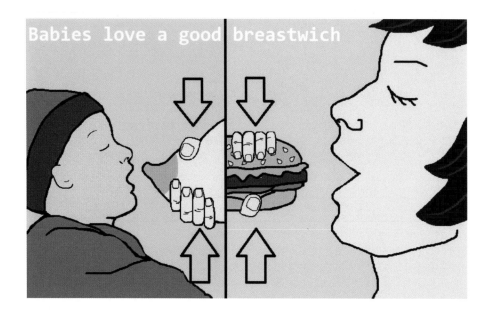

Babies love a good breastwich

In whatever breastfeeding position you choose, as long as your baby is in a good drinking position and is able to get as big a bite of your "breast sandwich" as possible, you're on the right track.

Now on to latching your baby!

Latching on in the "cross-cradle" position.

Step One:

Grip your baby in your dominant hand, and turn her body in towards you, belly-to-belly.

★ *Note: Your four fingers support the weight of your baby's head, and your palm wraps around her shoulder blades. Give your baby's butt a hug against your body, so that she is very close to you and feels secure.*

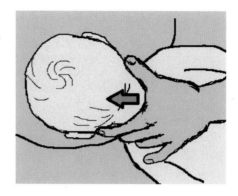

Step Two:

Align your baby so that her chin is touching your breast and your nipple is across from her nose.

★ *Note: Your baby's neck should be slightly extended, putting her in to that well aligned "drinking position" we discussed earlier.*

Step Three:

Grab your breast from underneath, about an inch or two back from your nipple, in a "U" shape.

★ *Note: Many women have an instinct to hold their breast, but they default to a "C"-shaped hold. When the baby is held in the cradle or cross-cradle position, the "C" hold squishes the breast into a "breast taco" instead of the desired "breast sandwich." In other words, the breast and the baby's mouth aren't lined up; the breast is squished vertically while the baby's mouth is horizontal. Think about trying to take a big bite of a hard shelled taco without turning your head sideways. It's not happening. But if you flip your hand to a "U" shape, the "breast burger" feast can commence.*

THE "C" HOLD

Used with upright football hold, side lying, and laid back positions

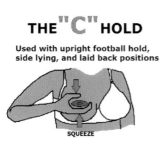

SQUEEZE

THE "U" HOLD

Used with cradle and cross cradle positions

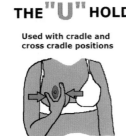

THE WHEEL OF TEARS

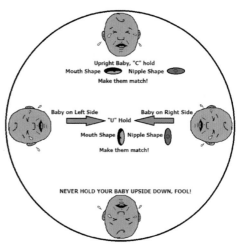

Put an end to the stress of getting that hangry child to latch! Follow the wheel of tears to know how to hold your breast when feeding your baby, and watch as those frowns turn **UPSIDE DOWN!**

Step Four:
Wait for your baby to open her mouth as widely as she can.

★ **Note:** *Think of your putting her into this position as a dinner invitation. If baby is interested in accepting, she will open her mouth widely as if to say, "Why thank you, I would be de-LIGHTED to join you for this milk fest." And when I say "widely," I mean WIDELY. When she looks like she is yawning, or about to start singing an opera, she is opening as widely as she can and it's time for you to make your move.*

And if she doesn't open? If she's just staring blankly at your boob? Well, she just refused your dinner invite. Why? Because she's lazy? Because she wants to make you mad? Because she's a little rebel baby with no respect for authority?

I sure hope not. If the above guesses are true, breastfeeding issues are the least of your worries. The reason most babies refuse a dinner invite is that they are simply not hungry. Or, perhaps they *are* hungry, but something else is going on in their bodies that needs to be dealt with before the meal. For newborns, the "something else" includes pooing, peeing, burping, farting or spitting up. Aren't babies fun?

But when you went through all the trouble of getting your baby ready for dinner and she has the audacity to refuse your invite, you're really going to feel like shoving your breast in to her mouth. Resist the temptation! Some babies who keep having nipples jammed into their mouths start refusing to latch altogether.

If your baby snubs your dinner invite, your best bet is to hold her skin-to-skin, wait for her to show hunger cues (which we'll talk about later), and then try again.

Call your pediatrician if your baby isn't eating well at least eight times in 24 hours.

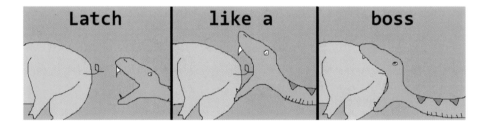

Step Five:
Bring your baby onto your breast with a quick push to her shoulder blades.

★ **Note:** *Because her chin is already against your breast, it's just a matter of bringing her wide-opened upper lip up and over your nipple (remember how you got up and over the too-big sandwich?).*

A fatal flaw occurs when mom acts too timidly during this part of the latch. A timid mom moves slowly and tentatively because she's afraid of damaging her seemingly fragile baby. But what this mother is forgetting is that her delicate little flower was just pushed, pulled, crammed, crushed and squeezed into the world in a fairly "extreme vagina sports" kind of way. Therefore, as long as you are adequately supporting her head and neck, your baby can definitely handle an assertive push to the shoulder blades.

Now hopefully, you have gotten baby on and she has started sucking. Because you started out with your nipple to her nose, more of your areola should be covered by her lower jaw than her upper lip. If you had x-ray glasses that could look through your baby's cheek, you would see your nipple all the way up in the roof of her mouth.

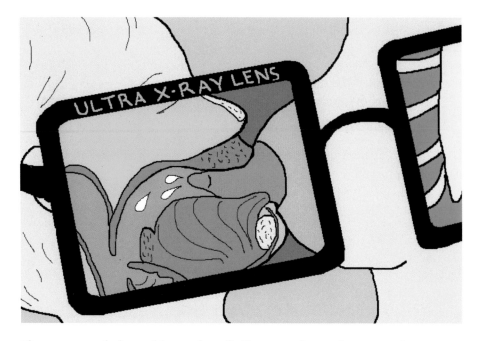

If you see your baby sucking and are feeling a gentle tugging at your breast, congrats, you've done it!

If you are grinding your teeth and saying "Ow, ow ow!" then something isn't right. You'll need to unlatch your baby by inserting your finger into her mouth to break the suction, and then return to Step 2.

When your baby is done feeding, notice the shape of your nipple when it comes out of her mouth. It should be nice and round and somewhat elongated. If it is squashed or pinched in any way, this is a sign your baby needs to be latched on more deeply.

Latching is a skill that takes time and practice. Be patient with yourself and with your baby. Shoot for the perfect latch every time you breastfeed and you will both be pros in no time!

Call a lactation consultant for help if you are having trouble getting comfortable.

Other positions.

We talked about laid-back positioning to achieve a baby-led latch and the cross-cradle position for ease of learning a mom-led latch. But of course there are other ways to do this. If your baby is drinking and you are comfortable, then your positioning is right...no matter what it looks like.

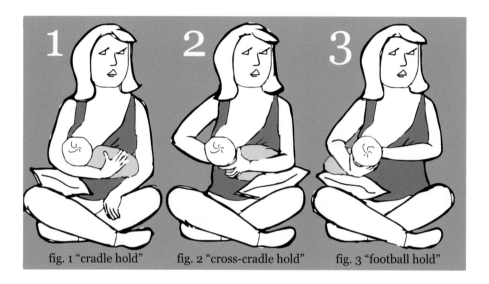

fig. 1 "cradle hold"   fig. 2 "cross-cradle hold"   fig. 3 "football hold"

Here are some standard breastfeeding positions:

Cradle: In this hold, baby's head is in the crook of your arm, and you hold their butt against your body with your hand. As you will see when you try it, latching on a big floppy head using your elbow tends to be trickier than using your hand. The good news is that once baby has better head control, this position gets easier. You could also latch your baby on in a cross-cradle position, and then switch to a cradle hold once you feel like the latch is solid.

Football: Guess what? If you know how to do the cross-cradle hold, you know how to do the football hold, too! Woo-hoo! Start in the cross-cradle position and then swing your baby around your front to the opposite breast. When their chin is touching the breast and their nose is lined up with your nipple, they're in the right place. Just like with the cross-cradle hold, wait until they open wide, and then give a big push on by the shoulderblades.

Side-Lying: This is where you and baby are lying down, facing each other. To try it out, lie down on the center of a firm mattress that's covered with a tight fitting sheet. There shouldn't be any pillows or blankets near your baby, and no risk of your baby falling off the bed.

Place your baby on their side, facing you, with their nose lined up to your nipple. Your knees will be slightly drawn up so that your body makes a "C" shape around the baby. The arm you're lying on will help latch your baby and the "on-top" arm will be in control of your breast. Wait until your baby opens wide, and then hug them in close to latch.

Like the cradle hold, this position tends to get easier as your baby gains head control. Side lying is a good position if you've had a C-section, or if you're just feeling the urge to lie down with your baby.

If you feel in danger of falling asleep, set an alarm for the length of the feed. That way, if you do fall asleep, your alarm will wake you and you can put your baby back into their safe sleep space.

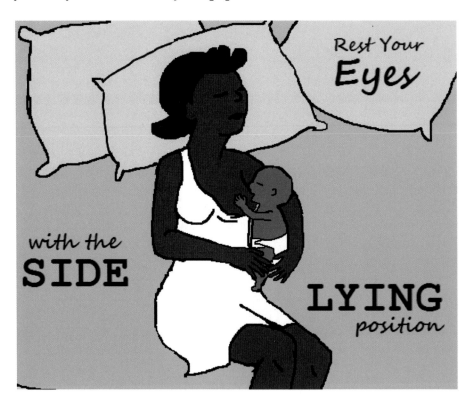

There is no harm in experimenting with new holds! Remember, if it's comfortable and baby's getting milk, it's right.

When to unlatch.

I've worked with many moms who struggle to latch their babies. After what seems like an eternity of frustration, struggling and crying (and sometimes the baby is crying too, ha-ha), the baby finally latches on. And even though this latch hurts, as in, mom's toes are curling in pain - she rejoices, "Glory Hallelujah, he's on!"

Unlatching her baby *on purpose* at this point seems laughable, and so the baby stays attached. Mom will suffer through the nipple pain if it means that her baby is eating.

But this mom is actually making things worse for both her...*and* her baby.

First, her baby is not getting as much milk as he could were he well attached. Second, her breasts are not getting drained well, which down-regulates her milk supply (we'll learn more about milk supply later) and causes the baby to be hungry more often. And third, her nipples are going to become painfully sore, which makes a hungry-all-the-time baby a terrible fate that can easily hasten the end of breastfeeding.

So if you find yourself in a situation where breastfeeding hurts, please un-latch your baby!

And don't just rip him off of your breast. Your baby is vacuumed sealed to your breast when he's latched, and if you just pull him back to take him off, your nipple's going to be coming along for the ride, being stretched and pinched before baby's dismount. Ouch!

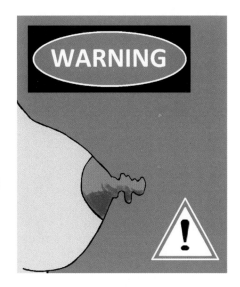

To unlatch your baby without causing nipple damage, make a fish-hook shape with your clean finger. Insert this into the corner of the baby's mouth to break the suction and now he'll easily slide off the breast.

Your nipples thank you in advance.

PART THREE: MAKING MILK

How it works.

Making milk comes down to a simple case of demand and supply. That's right, in the case of breastfeeding, the **demand comes first**, and the supply follows.

As soon as your baby is born, your milk making hormones perk up and say, "Congrats on getting the baby out! Tight fit, huh? Now let's get down to business. What would you like me to do? Make milk? Or not make milk? Cause I can go either way here, the choice is yours."

Anytime your baby breastfeeds (or you pump), the hormones send a message to your brain, **"MAKE MILK!"** And with every suck, that message is strengthened, "make milk, make milk, make milk!"

Therefore, if your baby is nursing a lot, more milk will result.

Higher demand from baby (or pump) = higher supply.

And the reverse is true as well. If your baby isn't being put to breast often, less milk will result.

Lower demand = lower supply.

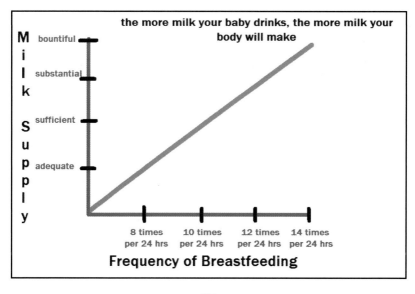

You will hear many people tell you that you can expect your milk "to come in" around day three post-partum. Which may make you wonder what the heck your baby's been eating in the meantime.

But never fear! Your body has been making **colostrum** (which is just a fancy word for the first milk your baby drinks) since about 16 weeks of pregnancy, and so you already have plenty of food available when your baby is born. Colostrum is small in volume, but tends to be enough to satisfy baby during the first few days. It is thicker than "mature" milk, and is usually a yellowish or clear color.

As your baby breastfeeds and the "**MAKE MILK**" message gets stronger and stronger, your body responds by producing more and more milk. The first few days of breastfeeding set up your milk supply for the entire length of your breastfeeding relationship. So put your baby to the breast early and often!

Engorgement.

Around day three, as your milk supply starts noticeably ramping up, your breasts will begin to feel full. This is normal, and a good sign that your baby and your body are doing what they are supposed to. Many moms (and let's face it, their partners) admire the new full, rounded and perky boobs that this baby has created. However, sometimes breasts become a little *too* full. Think bowling balls on steroids full. This over-fullness is called engorgement, and it's uncomfortable. But if you follow the below tips, you can expect it to get better within about a day or two.

To help with the discomfort of engorgement:

☑ **DO:** Nurse your baby whenever she tells you she's hungry, and at least eight times in 24 hours.

☑ **DO:** Place cold packs on your breasts between feedings.

☑ **DO:** Talk to your doctor about taking ibuprofen. Taking ibuprofen around the clock helps with the swelling and inflammation of engorgement, and is considered very safe for most breastfeeding mothers.

☑ **DO:** Use your pump or hand express for just a minute or two between feedings to take the edge off of any uncomfortable fullness.

☒ **DO NOT:** Pump to drain your breasts. Remember that milk making is all about demand and supply. The more milk you take out, the more milk your body will make to replace it. So pumping for more than just a few minutes will actually make your bowling ball boob problem worse.

☒ **DO NOT:** Use heat on your breasts for long periods. Heat increases blood flow to an area, and so it can worsen any swelling and inflammation. Heat on your breasts for just a minute or two right before a feeding may help your milk flow, but only use it if you need to.

☒ **DO NOT:** Suddenly quit breastfeeding because you decide it's for the dogs. Leaving your breasts full of milk can cause potential problems like plugged ducts and infections (mastitis). If you decide you want to stop breastfeeding, call a lactation consultant to help you wean in a way that lowers your risk for boob problems.

Call your doctor and a lactation consultant if along with the engorgement you notice painful breast lumps, flu-like symptoms, redness and/or streaking in your breasts, or a fever.

PART FOUR: BABY FEEDING

How often does your baby need to eat?

In order to make sure your milk increases in volume, to maintain your supply, and to ensure your baby is getting enough, you need to breastfeed at least eight times every 24 hours. Most babies will eat between 8-12 times a day.

Your baby isn't going to be eating on a regular schedule, and you need to be okay with that. It would be amazing if your baby ate every three hours on the dot. You could schedule meals, showers, go out, and make time for.... other adult activities. But your baby is not a robot, and just like the rest of us humans, will not eat the same amount at the same time every day.

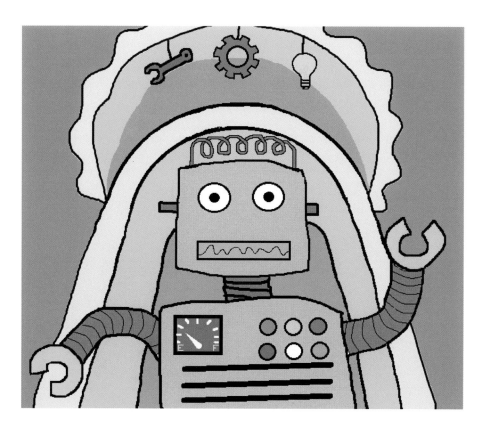

Hunger cues.

So how will you know when to feed your baby? Luckily, babies are born with fantastic communication skills and you'll never need to guess if they're hungry or not. From the moment they're born, they'll tell you:

Early Hunger Cues start with your baby squirming and opening and closing their mouth like a little baby bird. They will bring their hands to their mouth, and suck on them in a cute and happy manner. You'll see them turning their opened mouth towards your breast. Or should I say, you'll see them turning their mouth towards ANY breast that happens to be attached to the person holding them. This includes Grampa, Bill the next-door neighbor, and Uncle Ted.

Later Hunger Cues include whining, furiously frantic hand sucking, punching, kicking and head butting. Yup, you heard me right. Of course these are only *baby* karate moves, and so you'll survive this assault being no worse for the wear.

Hangry Hunger Cues include crying, back arching, and your baby thrashing their head around like a shark on the hunt.

So here's your game plan: Watch for baby's early hunger cues, and get them to the breast as quickly as possible. If you miss these early cues, and baby turns into the hangry shark, you'll need to modify your plan as hangry sharks don't latch on easily. Your best bet is to remove your baby from the breast, calm them down and then try again.

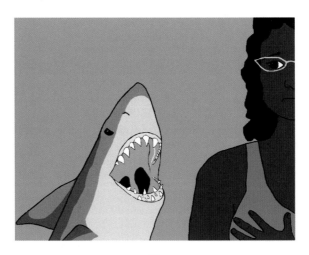

Three different sucks.

When baby is breastfeeding, he will show you three different types of sucks during different points in the feeding.

The first kind of suck is a **stimulating suck** that triggers milk flow. Breastfeeding moms don't walk around with milk continually pouring out of their breasts (which is such an evolutionary win when you think about it, am I right?). There is an ON/OFF switch in your brain, and your baby's stimulating suck controls it.

When baby first comes onto the breast, this relatively shallow yet rapid fire sucking sends a hormonal message to your brain saying, " HEY! I'm here and I'm hungry, turn the milk on!" This signal makes your milk start to flow or "let down."

As your baby begins to drink, you'll notice him switch to the second type of suck, a deeper, slower, wide and rhythmic suck called a **nutritive suck**. When you see this type of sucking, it is a good sign that your baby is actively eating. The whole side of his jaw moves rhythmically, and you'll see his chin taking big dips up and down. If you notice a slight pause when his chin drops and listen closely, you might hear him swallowing.

Your baby will probably switch back and forth between stimulating sucks and nutritive sucks during a feed. When the flow of milk slows, baby will start his stimulating sucking back up, which tells your brain, "HEY! I'm still here and still hungry, send more milk!"

As the feeding slows down and baby becomes satisfied, he may detach himself from the breast, or he may stay attached and change his suck to the third type: a gentle, fluttery and more sporadic suck known as a **non-nutritive suck**. When you see this, your baby is most likely not getting a lot of milk, and is just chillaxin' at the breast. You may notice your baby doing this non-nutritive sucking in his sleep, too!

It's important to be able to identify which suck your baby is using at any point during a feed, so that you can tell when to switch sides and when the feeding is over.

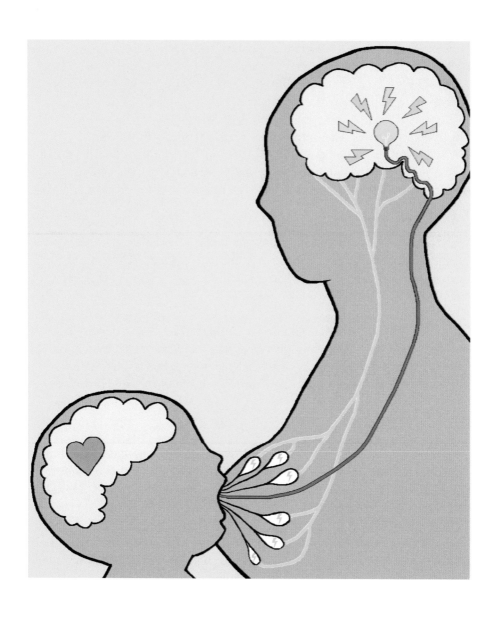

Switching sides.

A very common question is, "How do I know when it's time to switch sides?" You may have heard that you need to time feedings: ten minutes on one side, ten minutes on the other. But that's not the greatest way to make sure a baby is getting enough to eat. What if baby latches and goes to town eating, and is still showing you active nutritive sucking at the ten minute mark? Should you switch her just because ten minutes is up? Or what if she feeds well for seven minutes, pops off and won't relatch? Should you try and force her back on to that boob? Or is it time to switch?

Do you see how a timed feeding might cause confusion?

A better way to figure out when to switch sides is by watching your baby instead of the clock. If baby gets on the first side and is using those wide rhythmic nutritive sucks, you should keep her there for as long as she's doing that. She may stay on the first side for five minutes, ten, 15 or 20.

The time it takes her to finish the first breast will depend upon a variety of things including your milk supply at that moment, as well as how tired and hungry she is. So even though the time spent on the first breast may change at every feeding, you'll always know when it's time to switch because you'll know when your breast is mostly empty.

Ok, so then how do you know when your breast is mostly empty?

Well, there are a few ways:

- One way is to watch your baby's sucking pattern. Most babies appear very active at the beginning of a feed. You'll see a lot of switching between stimulating and nutritive sucking without many pauses. As the breast empties and her tummy fills, your baby may appear to lose steam. She'll take longer and longer pauses in between the nutritive sucking bursts, and may start to add some non-nutritive sucking into the mix. This means your breast is mostly empty and it's time to switch sides.

- Another good sign that your breast is mostly empty and it's time to switch is that it was firm and perky when the feeding began and now feels soft and squishy.

- You can use breast compressions to make sure your breast is mostly empty and it's time to switch. A breast compression is just what it sounds like - you squeeze your boob. When baby starts to slow down on her sucking, give your breast a squeeze and watch her response. If she starts showing wide rhythmic sucking again, hold that squeeze until she's stopped. Then move your hand to a new spot on your breast. Wait for your baby to start sucking again, and squeeze your boob again. Once baby no longer responds to the squeezes, you'll know that breast is pretty empty and it's time to switch sides.

Always offer the second side. Baby may or may not take it, but always offer. If baby is interested in the second breast, you'll see things play out in much the same way they did on the first breast. Baby will drink actively for a bit, and then appear to gradually lose steam. When baby removes herself from the breast, is only showing non-nutritive sucking, or falls asleep, the feeding is finished.

A note on "mostly empty" breasts:
A lactating breast is never *truly* empty. As long as there is a baby or a pump on that breast asking for milk, the hormones are flowing to your brain and your body will respond by making more milk. If you pump, you can watch your breasts "let down" milk several times during a pumping session. When you start, the milk will flow steadily, and then it will slow down or even stop...but if you keep the pump running, you will see milk flowing again within a few minutes. Cool, huh?

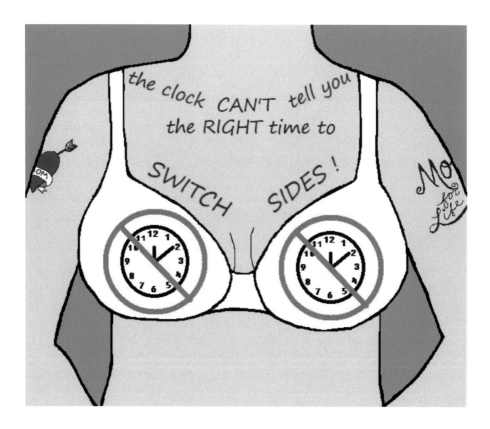

How do you know this is working?

You're now a few days into breastfeeding your baby. You don't feel super clumsy anymore, the latch is comfortable, and your baby is eating 8-12 times every 24 hours. Things seem great!

And they probably are.

But I know moms, and I know the overwhelming feeling of responsibility that comes with bringing your baby home and literally having their life depend on you. When you start wondering if they are getting enough to eat the anxiety can easily take over.

In your moments of doubt, you may be tempted to grab a bottle of formula, or to pump and bottle feed, so that you can measure baby's intake. But if your goal is exclusive breastfeeding, and you know how to tell your baby is getting enough *without* measuring the milk, you can feel more confident about keeping them solely on the boob.

There are four good ways to know that breastfeeding is working well and that your baby is thriving:

1. Count baby's diapers. One wet and one poo diaper on day one. Two and two on day two. Three and three on day three. Four and four on day four. On day five and beyond, you will want to see six or more wet diapers and four poos during every 24-hour cycle (a poo needs to be as big as a quarter for it to count).

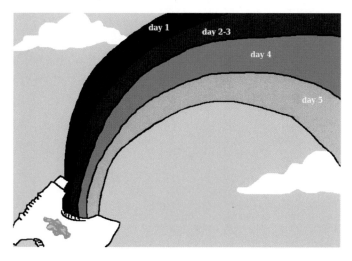

Also notice the color and texture changes of the poos. They will start out a thick sticky blackish color (called "meconium"), thin out a bit and turn greenish around day three and then be seedy and yellow with a mustardy texture by day five. If your diapers are adding up and changing color as expected, baby is getting enough milk!

2. Watch baby's behavior. Does baby show hunger cues before feeding, wide rhythmic sucking during a feeding and then look satisfied and relaxed at the end? Is he giving you at least a couple of two or three hour stretches in a day of happy and relaxed behavior? If you've answered "yes," these are great signs that baby is getting enough!

3. Monitor baby's weight. Most babies lose weight in the first few days of life. This is expected. They are pooing and peeing up a storm, but they are not eating large amounts yet. A 5-7% loss is considered normal. Anything higher than this and you should get some feeding help from a lactation consultant. Once your mature milk comes in around day three, your baby should start putting on about 2/3 of an ounce to one ounce every day. Your pediatrician will help you keep track. If baby's weight gain is on target, you're doing great!

4. Pay attention to your breasts. Did your breasts get bigger during pregnancy? Did you notice your breasts becoming more round and perky around day three after birth? Do your breasts feel firmer at the start of a feeding and softer once baby has nursed? If so, these are more good signs that your body is doing what it's supposed to and your baby is getting enough.

If any of the above seem off, your baby *might not* be getting enough. If you are not getting the diapers you should, if baby is crying and showing hunger cues around the clock despite frequent feeds, if he isn't gaining weight well, if you never felt breast changes, or if you feel like something is just not right, then it's time to get help. Call the pediatrician to make sure your baby is getting enough to eat... and then contact a lactation consultant to figure out how to get breastfeeding on track.

A note on bottles and pacifiers:

In general, if all is going well, try to focus on giving your baby only your nipple and only your milk until breastfeeding is well established (this usually doesn't happen before the two week mark). That being said, there are times when moms need to or choose to use pacifiers, bottles and formula before breastfeeding is going well, and that's totally cool. A pacifier is a tool. A bottle is a tool. Formula is a tool. They are all in your breastfeeding toolbelt. You may need to use them in order to keep your baby fed and your sanity intact while you figure out how to make breastfeeding work.

A baby getting breastmilk exclusively from the breast never trumps your physical, mental or emotional health.You are an equal part of the breastfeeding relationship and **YOU MATTER**! Get some help from a lactation consultant if you feel as though things are not going smoothly, and she will help you use the tools available in a way that helps you meet your baby feeding goals.

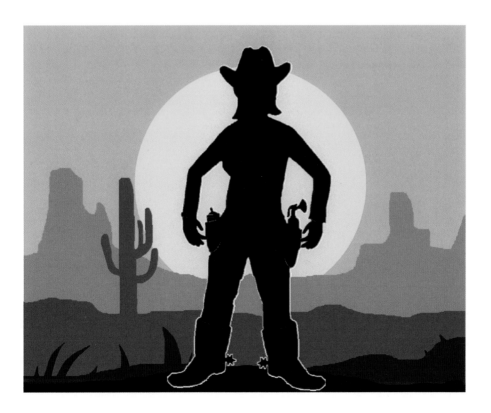

CONCLUSION

Hooray! We've reached the end of Breastfeeding 101. You now have basic breastfeeding knowledge, and hopefully feel more prepared for your upcoming adventures in baby feeding.

Remember that even though you are doing everything you can to prepare, breastfeeding will most likely still pose some challenges. However, hard work, dedication, and patience tend to pay off after a few weeks and result in an easy, relaxing, and fun breastfeeding relationship. And this is a beautiful thing!

But you know what's even more beautiful? The love that a mother has for her child, regardless of how he is fed. Good parenting is not defined by bottles or boobs, cloth or disposable diapers, strollers or baby carriers, or non-GMO organic cotton crib sheets. Good parenting is about whether or not your child feels your love. Period. And if he does, then no matter how you're going about baby feeding and parenting in general...you're doing it right!

I wish you luck, love and happy nipples on your baby feeding adventure!

THE END

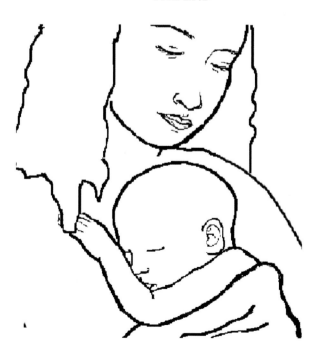

41

Made in the USA
Columbia, SC
20 December 2020

28852842R10024